Getting Ready for Dialysis: What You Need to Know

by Deepak Mittal, MD

Getting Ready for Dialysis:
What You Need to Know

Copyright © 2015 by Deepak Mittal

Cover by: Valerie Mellema

Book Website
www.kdcflorence.com
Email: nkydoc@gmail.com

Office Location:
47 Cavalier Blvd. Suite #120
Florence, KY 41042
(859) 757-4353

Printed in U.S.A

Dedication

To my parents Pushpa Mittal and K C Mittal, my wife Bahar and kids Amisha Ria and Rishi.

Table of Contents

Introduction..9
Chapter 1 11
My Doctor Said I Need Dialysis..............................11
Chapter 2 13
Dialysis Options 13
Chapter 3 17
Types of Dialysis Access 17
Chapter 4 21
What to Expect at the HD Clinic 21
Chapter 5 25
The Home Dialysis Clinic.......................................25
Chapter 6 27
Role of the Dietician 27
Chapter 7 31
The Best Outcomes 31
Chapter 8 33
The Role of the Social Worker 33
Chapter 9 35
Bone Health 35
Chapter 10...37
Preventing Infections 37
Chapter 11...39
Networking with Other Patients.............................39
Chapter 12...41
Traveling When You Are on Dialysis 41
Chapter 13...45
When Should I Call the Doctor? 45
Chapter 14...47
Am I a Transplant Candidate? 47
Chapter 15...51
Special Olympics...51

Chapter 16..53

Do You Have High Cholesterol?..53

Chapter 17..57

Working and Dialysis 57

Chapter 18..59

Family Fatigue 59

Chapter 19..63

Dealing with Depression 63

Chapter 20..65

American Kidney Fund and Renal Network 65

Chapter 21..67

Getting Help with Prescription Costs................................67

Chapter 22..69

Frequently Asked Questions..69

Chapter 23..73

Becoming a Star Patient 73

Chapter 24..75

Do I Need Handicap Parking?...75

Chapter 25..77

My Nurse Was Rude!...77

Chapter 26..79

Learning the Lingo - Your Quick and Simple Glossary 79

Conclusion..83

About the Author 85

Introduction

Welcome to the patient guide! We know that you probably have quite a few questions about dialysis as well as what exactly it will mean for you, and that's the goal of this book - to give you a better understanding of your situation, what you can expect with dialysis, and how you can keep your quality of life as good as possible.

Of course, you might not know me very well at this point. You've just started coming into the clinic, and you might want a little more info on who I am and where I am coming from.

Who Am I and Why Did I Write This Book?

When I was just a child, I had family members who were on dialysis. My aunt would go to dialysis three times each week. I also cared for my sister who suffered from nephritis. You see, since I was quite young, I had a connection to kidney disease, and I was determined that I needed to do something to help as many people as I could.

I studied hard, keeping my eyes on the goal of becoming a doctor, and then specializing in nephrology. I studied at Government Medical College Patiala, the All India Institute of Medical Sciences, and the University of Louisville School of Medicine to gain the knowledge needed to help patients just like you.

Today, I work closely with Fresenius Dialysis, and I am their Medical Director at their Edgewood and Boone County Dialysis Centers. And that's how we came to meet.

Now that you know a little bit more about me and why I am so passionate about helping patients with kidney disease and who go on dialysis, it's time to go forward and get into the bulk of this book, namely helping you.

Throughout the course of this book, we'll be covering topics that are likely of high interest to you - your options with dialysis, what you can expect when you come into the clinic, home dialysis, traveling, working, transplants, and much more. Now, let's get into it!

Chapter 1

My Doctor Said I Need Dialysis

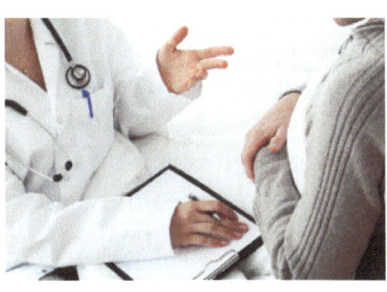

Your health is of the utmost concern for you as well as for us, and it is entirely understandable and natural that you have more than a healthy dose of fear when it comes to the dreaded "D" word: dialysis. No one welcomes the news of kidney failure and the need to go on dialysis. It's important that you take the time to gain a better understanding of what you will experience and to learn ways to make the process and the news easier to bear. That's the goal of this book - to provide you with the answers you need as well as to help allay some of the worry that you are feeling right now.

The Feelings Are Natural

Fear is one of the most natural and common reactions to learning that you will need to start undergoing dialysis treatment. It's a brand new experience, and you likely have very little idea of what will be happening to you and what the process will be like. You may have little to no knowledge or understanding of the procedures or of what you will need to do. Most people don't until they've experienced it or had a loved one on dialysis.

You feel nervous and ill-prepared to deal with the situation. Many patients feel as though dialysis means their life is over and that they will never again be able to do the things that they once loved. Knowledge can help to reduce these fears.

Ask Questions

One of the most important things you can do to help combat

your fear is to ask questions and clear away the mystery surrounding your condition and dialysis. Your first worries are whether you are dying and how long you have to live. You want to know about how dialysis works and what types of things you will need to change in your life. Do you need to have peritoneal dialysis or can you do home dialysis? How often will you even need to do dialysis? Perhaps you are wondering whether you might be able to get a transplant. Is it possible to reverse the problem and restore normal kidney function?

While this book will answer many of the questions that you have, you certainly shouldn't stop there. The doctor and the healthcare staff want to make sure you understand every step of the process and everything you need to do to improve your condition as much as possible.

No matter what type of questions you have, and no matter how trivial they might seem to you, make sure that you ask them. No matter what they are, the staff should always do their very best to provide you with answers.

The Good News

You might be thinking that there is no good news if you discover you will need to go on dialysis. That's not the case, at least not in today's modern medical world. Fortunately, dialysis has come a long way in the past couple of decades, and it's no longer quite as scary and debilitating as it once was. It's not going to be a walk in the park, but thanks to the improvements in technology, as well as the growing education and support options available, things are looking much brighter.

Over the remainder of this book, we'll be doing our very best to provide you with answers to many of the questions that you have right now, and even some answers to questions you didn't know you had. Of course, if you have any other concerns or questions that we don't cover here, be sure to ask them. We'll find the answers you need.

Chapter 2

Dialysis Options

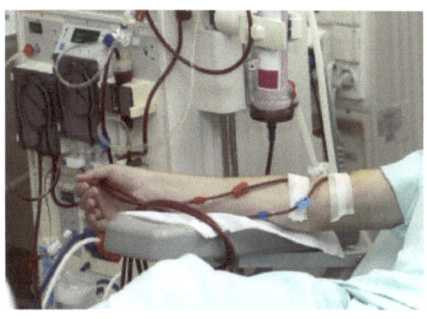

After receiving your diagnosis, if it appears as though dialysis might be the next step, it is important that you remain as proactive as possible. This means you should start to learn more about the options available to you. In general, you will be able to choose between three options, but not all of these options are going to be right for all patients, naturally. Let's look at the possibilities available.

More than 2.5 million people in the world go through dialysis on a daily basis, so you are not alone, no matter how frightened you might feel when you realize you will need to have dialysis. You are able to do the treatments at home or in a clinic, and it can help to ensure that you do not continue to damage your kidneys.

Dialysis in the Center

The majority of the patients who have kidney failure will need to come into the clinic several times per week (three or four, usually) in order to receive their hemodialysis treatment. The dialysis machine will pump the blood from a shunt in your lower arm into a dialyzer, which is essentially an "artificial kidney."

The machine will then filter the waste from the blood, just as the kidneys would do when functioning normally. It has anticoagulants in the dialysis fluid to ensure the blood does not clot. After the waste is removed from the blood, the blood is then returned to the body.

Dialysis requires that a large amount of blood goes through

the machine. It's not possible to use the veins alone, as they don't carry as much blood as needed, and it's not possible to use the arteries alone because they pump the blood at too high a rate.

Home Dialysis (Peritoneal Dialysis)

Peritoneal dialysis is very different, and some patients may qualify for this type of procedure. The peritoneum, which is the name for the natural lining in the abdominal cavity, will actually filter the blood. It works in a fashion that's very similar to the dialyzer mentioned above. Currently, a small number of patients who are suffering from kidney failure (around 270,000 out of 2.5 million) choose this type of treatment. One of the benefits of the treatment is that patients are able to do it at home, so they will not have to come into the clinic.

Currently, there are several options when it comes to peritoneal dialysis. The first is called CAPD, or Continuous Ambulatory Peritoneal Dialysis. With this type of treatment, you will manually change out their dialysis solution several times each day - generally four or five. It's a relatively simple bag system and it is easy for you or for your caretakers to learn. We'll discuss the details of how the system works in the next chapter.

The second option is APD, Automatic Peritoneal Dialysis. This option features a dialysis machine that will handle the exchange of the old dialysis solution for new, and it's popular as an overnight treatment. Again, the benefit is that you will be able to handle this type of treatment by yourself. This allows you to have far more freedom when it comes to your social life and their work life. You will not have to worry about making it to the clinic for the dialysis treatment.

There is one more potential option that you may be able to find in some locations, and that is home hemodialysis using a Fresenius K machine or NxStage System One. It's a machine that you can use at home, providing you with greater control over when you go through dialysis. Again, these types of home dialysis will help you to regain some semblance of a normal life, allowing you to do the things you want to do and need to do again.

Kidney Transplant

Another one of the options that may be a viable one for some patients is a kidney transplant. However, this is not a solution for everyone, and not everyone will be a good candidate for a transplant. Essentially, this surgical procedure will take a kidney from a deceased donor, or from a live person, and replace one of your own kidneys. One of the things that you will have to keep in mind is that there is a limited supply of donor kidneys available, and the waitlist tends to be rather long.

We will be covering this in detail in Chapter 14, so you can get a better idea of whether you might be a suitable donor or not. As always, when you have questions about your condition, and if you want to know more about transplants, speak with your physician.

Enroll in the Options Class

You probably have quite a few more questions about your dialysis options, don't you? It's natural, and it's great that you are doing as we suggested earlier and are taking an active role in understanding your options and getting answers.

Ask your nephrologist about enrolling in the next Options Class. These classes are taught by nurses who will provide one-on-one training, as well as videos to help you get a better understanding of what is available to you. They will be able to go over all of your options with you and help you determine which will be the best solution for your needs.

Chapter 3
Types of Dialysis Access

Access, or the way in which the dialysis procedure and solution are performed, is extremely important to understand. In the last chapter, we discussed the basics of the different option in dialysis, and here, we'll be going into more detail on what you can expect with the different types of dialysis in the clinic and at home.

In-Center Dialysis

In order to obtain the blood in a safe manner, and to ensure that enough blood is flowing through the dialysis machine, the patient will need to have a vascular access shunt placed in the lower arm. This is created by the doctor's during a simple procedure where they join a vein and an artery, described as a fistula. It has no negative effects on the circulation, but it will make access to the blood easier for dialysis.

There is only a very small incision when the doctor connects the vein and the artery, but it will generally take between six and eight weeks to heal properly. In most cases, this is best done when you are in stage-four kidney disease.

If for some reason the vein is not good, the surgeon will do what is called a graft. They add a plastic device that will act as the connector between the vein and the artery. One of the benefits of this procedure is that it will typically only take about two weeks to heal. However, there is a potential downside, as these can sometimes clog. Surgeons will generally prefer to create the fistula.

If the dialysis is needed sooner than two to six weeks, it is possible to use a catheter placed into one of the body's larger blood vessels. These are placed into the body in a vein in the neck, just below your clavicle. It is usually placed on the right side.

However, this is only a temporary solution, and the patient will likely need to receive a shunt eventually. This is something you will want to discuss with your healthcare professionals.

Something to note about these procedures is that since they are surgical procedures, even though they are relatively minor, there is always a chance for infection. We'll be covering this in depth in Chapter 10.

Your nurse will be able to provide you with detailed instructions on how to prevent infection and how to care for an infection if it starts. In addition, the nurse will be able to provide you with tips and guidelines on how to make sure the incision, shunt, and more are safe, including all of the water precautions you need to take.

For Home Dialysis Patients

With this type of treatment, the doctors will place a catheter into the abdominal cavity. The dialysis solution is then added to the abdominal cavity via the catheter. 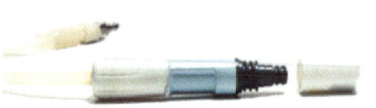 The blood is then filtered, with the toxins flowing into the solution. The glucose that's in the dialysis solution will pull water from the body as well, helping to remove more toxins. When the procedure is finished, the old, toxin-filled solution is removed through the catheter, and then a new solution is added.

It will generally take about two weeks for the catheter to mature in the body, and at that point, the medical staff will be able to provide training for you so you understand how to use the equipment and the solution. It might be a little intimidating when you are first starting, but it's really quite simple once you go through the training.

Once again, there is a chance of infection, so you do need to make sure you are taking the proper precautions. The training will help you understand how to keep everything as clean and sterile as possible so you can reduce your risk of developing an infection.

Make Sure You Understand the Training

Chances are good that you do not have any extensive medical training. This means that the idea of preventing infections, performing your own peritoneal dialysis, and undergoing all of these procedures is foreign to you. As we mentioned earlier in the book, fear and confusion are natural. We always do our best to allay your fears and to answer your questions. Always feel free to ask about what you need to do in order to remain as healthy as possible. We'll explain everything so you will understand every step of the procedure.

Chapter 4

What to Expect at the HD Clinic

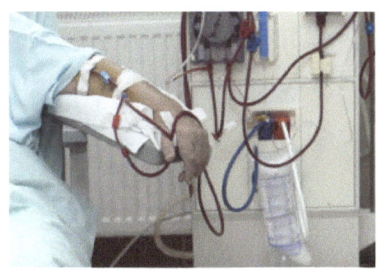

Now, let's look a bit deeper at what you can expect when you come into the clinic for hemodialysis for the first time. Knowing what is coming will certainly make the entire process much easier for you.

The First Steps

First, you want to make sure you get to the clinic early for your first and all of your subsequent dialysis treatments. This ensures that you are not rushing around at the last minute and that you will feel more relaxed and comfortable when you get into the treatment room.

When you get into the treatment room, the nurse will get you seated in the chair and will tell you everything that's going to happen during the treatment. By now, you should know if you have any questions about what's happening, feel free to ask the nurse. He or she will explain it all.

Here's a quick tip. You should consider bringing a blanket along with you so you will be comfortable in case you get cold. The temperature in the room is around 65 degrees. It's kept at this temperature to cut down on the risk of infection. Having a blanket will keep you warmer, and every little bit of added comfort helps. Of course, if you like it a bit cooler, the temperature will probably be perfect for you. It's better to have a blanket rather than dressing too warmly, as this will make it easier for you to regulate how warm you are.

Something else to keep in mind is that you will not be allowed to have family and friends with you in the dialysis treatment room. They are allowed to wait for you in the waiting room, though. Don't be nervous without them! You can meet other patients who are going through dialysis and speak with them. They can be a great source of encouragement and information. They have been through it and can let you know what it is like from a patient's perspective.

You can also take this time to learn the names of the staff, the social worker, and the dietician. Of course, during your first visit, chances are you will be nervous and you might not remember everyone's name. That's okay! As you get more comfortable and come to more treatment sessions, you will start to remember their names.

What Can You Do?

Most of the times, a dialysis treatment will take about four hours. One of the worries that some patients have is that they will be bored when they are going through the treatment. You will only be as bored as you allow yourself to be. You have quite a few things to do to help you keep busy while you are going through treatment.

You will be able to watch television, or read a book. It's a nice time to stock up on some reading material that you can bring along with you. You might even want to spend your time writing that novel or screenplay that you have been thinking of writing. Maybe you just want to get a little bit of sleep. In some of the centers, there are even iPads available. Talk with the staff about what types of items you are able to bring in with you when you are undergoing treatment.

As mentioned, there will be other patients in the clinic going through dialysis treatment as well. You can talk with them, share some recipes, and just get to know them a little bit better. In fact, high protein recipes are very popular among the patients, and they can let you know of some fantastic recipes that will be perfect for you.

In addition, you will have visits from the social worker to see how you are doing, as well as the nurse, who will perform foot checks and listen to your lungs. The nurse will also educate you on fluid intake. Something you will want to learn is your "dry weight." This weight, measured in kilograms rather than pounds, is checked both before and after the dialysis procedure.

The staff and the patients quickly become like family with one another, and you will start to feel very comfortable in no time. Everyone wants the best for you!

Chapter 5
The Home Dialysis Clinic

Perhaps you've decided to do the home peritoneal dialysis instead. This is a fantastic alternate option for traditional dialysis at the clinic. Patients who are still working will find that it's a fantastic option, even though it is currently much rarer than hemodialysis at the clinic.

If that's the case, you will need to have training on how to perform the procedures properly. At this point, some patients become worried that it will be too complex for them or their families to handle. That's not the case at all, though. Doctor's wouldn't allow this type of treatment if it were something that you couldn't do! All it takes is a little training.

For the most part, this type of dialysis is better for younger patients. Older patients will often have other illnesses, and that can make performing home dialysis on their own far more difficult. Talk with your doctor about whether you feel you are in a good position to have home dialysis.

The Training

The peritoneal dialysis training is actually quite simple, and it will only take between three and five days to complete. The nurse will train you in all aspects of the procedures. They will go over all of the various protocols and machines, and the fluids you will be using. You will learn how to operate the cycler as well. In the beginning, all of the new machines and terms might be confusing, but the nurse does a great job at breaking it all down so you can understand it.

You will learn how to handle any types of minor problems that might occur. These are rare, but having the knowledge of what to do will give you much more peace of mind. You can ask as many questions as you need so you understand the process completely. We work hard to ensure you are never lost or confused when it comes to these procedures.

Training for Others in the Family

Ideally, you will not be the only one in the family learning all of these procedures. It's best if you have several people, such as a spouse, a parent, an adult child, or a friend that can learn the process and procedures as well. This way, if you need some help or you are 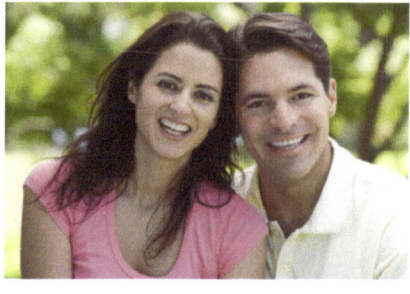 unable to do the tasks on your own for some reason, you have someone nearby who can provide a helpful and knowledgeable hand.

However, even though it's a good idea to have other people trained in helping you at home ... you might not actually need them, which is why so many patients are choosing peritoneal dialysis.

Remain Independent

One of the biggest benefits of peritoneal dialysis is that you don't actually need to have much family support when it comes to using the equipment. Most of our patients using this method find that they are quite capable of taking care of it all on their own. This allows them to have more freedom and independence, and they enjoy the fact that they don't have to ask family members to help them all the time.

Because of these benefits, we're finding that this is one of the fastest growing trends in this field today. We're proud to be able to offer this option for our patients, and it might be something that you want to consider. Please make sure you talk with us about whether you might be a good candidate for this option. While it might not be right for everyone, it might be right for you. We will let you know!

Chapter 6

Role of the Dietician

When you have kidney failure and you are going through dialysis, proper attention to your diet is extremely important. Too many patients who have kidney failure simply don't pay enough attention to the foods they are putting into their body. 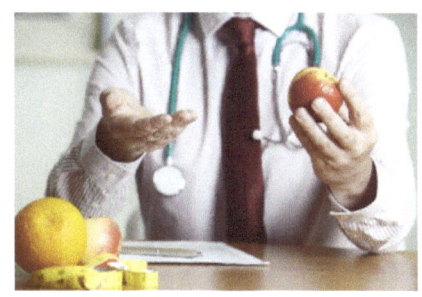 When you work with us, we look at the entire picture to provide you with the best possible results for your health, and that includes your nutrition.

Your dietician is one of the keys to your success. They will provide you with a variety of different recipes that you can try, and you can run some of your own recipes, and those you've collected, by the dietician. He or she will be able to help tailor a diet to your specific needs.

How Will the Dietician Help?

Some patients who are going through dialysis are diabetic as well, and this means that the dietary requirements are even more important. The dietician can ensure that you are eating the right foods and using the healthiest recipes to help with your condition.

Each month, we'll check your lab tests and will measure the phosphorous in your blood. The dietician will help you understand how to lower the phosphorous and to reach your goals. In addition, the doctor and the dietician might find that you need to take special medications called binders. This type of medication is specifically for controlling the level of phosphorous in the blood.

The labs will also check for the level of calcium in the blood, and the doctor and dietician will provide proper medications for regulation if needed. In addition, the dialysis machine can also help with excess calcium in the blood. The nurse will help you understand how this works.

Naturally, your cholesterol is important to watch as well. The foods the dietician tells you to eat, along with getting the right amount of mineral and vitamin supplementation can help with this substantially.

Importance of Protein in the Diet

One of the most important nutritional elements for someone going through dialysis is protein. If you do not have enough protein in the body, it means you will not be able to heal properly. You will not be able to fight infection effectively, and it can even be difficult to stop bleeding.

For those who suffer from chronic kidney disease, getting enough protein can be a real problem. It is also more difficult for the kidneys to remove protein waste when you are suffering from kidney failure. As you progress through the stages of kidney failure, it can become more difficult. When in the early stages of kidney failure, the doctors will often say to go on a low protein diet since the kidneys have trouble getting rid of the waste.

However, when you are on dialysis, this process takes care of filtering the protein waste, and that means you will need to increase the level of protein intake so you can get the benefits that it provides. Having a higher protein intake can ensure you get your needed protein, as well as amino acids.

It is important that you are eating the right types of protein. You will generally want to stay away from the fatty forms of protein, as this could raise your cholesterol. You will also want to avoid protein rich foods that are high in phosphorous. As we've discussed, you will want to keep these elements down. Some good options for protein that are low in fat and highly healthy include chicken breast, fish, and low-fat dairy products.

Your dietician can provide details on the protein intake that is right for your specific needs. The amount of protein you need will vary based on your stage of chronic kidney disease, your size, current healthy, and the lab results you get each month.

Collect Recipes

As we mentioned in the last chapter, it is quite common for patients who are going through dialysis treatment to start talking about food and sharing recipes. It's nice to share ones that you have and to take ideas from other patients. However, in the interest of your health, it is generally a good idea to speak with your dietician about the recipe before trying it. They can look over the ingredients and make sure it is right for you.

Remember, all patients are different, and you may have another condition that could make it unhealthy for you to eat certain foods. Running it by the dietician is a simple way to make sure you have a quality recipe that's actually going to be good for you!

Chapter 7
The Best Outcomes

Everyone wants to have the best possible outcome when undergoing dialysis treatment. We want the very best for you as well, and that's why we work hard to monitor your health. We consider the governmental guidelines and keep up with all of the studies that are highlighting the most important aspects of improving a patient's outcome. We implement this into your care so you can be as healthy as possible during your treatments and while you are at home.

What Helps to Improve Your Outcome?

One of the most common questions that people have when it comes to outcome improvement is just which elements are the most important. Studies have shown that several factors play vital roles:

- A good fistula
- No infection
- Controlled diet
- Adjustment to medications

We're able to help with each of these things. The doctors work hard to ensure that you have a good fistula so that it's easier process during the dialysis. The same holds true for those patients with a catheter that are doing their own dialysis treatments from home.

Proper care of the fistula and catheter area are essential when it comes to reducing the chance of getting an infection. In Chapter 10, we'll cover infections in depth. In the last chapter, we talked about the importance of having a dietician to help regulate your nutrition. These, along with taking the right medications, can really help to provide you with a better overall outcome.

The Monthly CQI Meetings

We hold a CQI (Continuous Quality Improvement) meeting each month. During these meetings, the doctor, nurse manager, dietician, and social workers gather to talk about the quality measures in use with all of our patients. Your goal is to become a "star patient" by meeting the quality indicators we have in place.

We discuss the patient's labs and markers each month. Some of the most important markers that we discuss include:

- Presence of fistula
- Phosphorous control
- Calcium control
- Hemoglobin control
- Improving albumin levels
- Control of fluid intake
- Avoiding fluid retention
- Control of blood pressure

We take what we learn from the CQI meeting and then implement it into your care plan. We do this to ensure that you are getting the best and proper treatment.

Chapter 8

The Role of the Social Worker

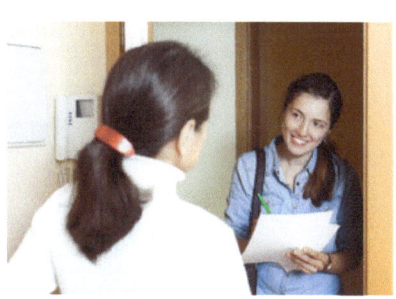

Many new patients do not understand just how important the social worker is when it comes to their wellbeing. They play a very important role in your support system and they will be a huge benefit to you and to your family. They act as an advocate for you, and they can help to communicate any needs that you might have to the rest of the medical staff.

What Does the Social Worker Do?

The social worker will create an assessment shortly after meeting you. They will ask a number of different questions during this time to get a better understanding of your health and any issues you might have that could play a role during your treatment.

Some might be a bit reticent to share this information at first, but you have to remember that the social worker is on your side and is working with you and the medical staff to make sure you are getting the best treatment possible. They have to understand your needs, so it is very important that you are honest when you are talking with the social worker and answering their questions.

How Can the Social Worker Help?

The social worker has a number of different roles. They will help you to adjust to life with kidney disease and all of the changes that going through dialysis can bring. They help to explain just how important it is to participate in the treatment and to follow the guidelines of the medical staff. In the last chapter, we touched on the fact that the social workers are also part of the monthly CQI meetings, which help to improve the patient outcomes.

They will help to provide you with more education and resources too, as well as any referrals you might need. They can help you to keep or find insurance coverage, and help you learn more about your rights and responsibilities. The social worker can help you get the medication you need through different programs, they can help to arrange transportation, and so much more. Many times, they will also evaluate you for rehabilitation services so you can get back to work.

Your social worker is a great resource, so make sure you take advantage of everything he or she is capable of offering. When you have questions, they can provide you with answers, and if they don't know the answer, they can find them out for you.

Chapter 9

Bone Health

How healthy are your bones? While you might not immediately understand how your kidneys could affect your bones, it's actually very simple. You need to have good phosphorous and calcium for your bones to be healthy. However, because the kidneys have trouble filtering, this often means that the calcium and phosphorous are wasted. That's why we perform the lab tests. If you have too much calcium and phosphorous in your results, it means you could have unhealthy bones, as these nutrients are being leached out of them.

Let's look at little deeper into calcium and phosphorus to see why they are important for your health.

What Is Calcium?

Calcium is a type of mineral that's found in the body. It and phosphorous help to keep the bones strong. Calcium is also important for powering the muscles and it is carried through the body via the blood system. It's typically found in green vegetables, as well as dairy products and eggs.

What Is Phosphorous?

Phosphorous is another mineral in the body and it helps to create a number of different biochemical reactions. You need to take in phosphorous from food sources, such as dairy products and nuts.

Kidney disease patients will suffer from something called PTH, or parathyroid hormone. As mentioned, this draws the calcium out of the bones when the calcium level in the blood drops. The high levels of calcium and phosphorous in your lab results means that your bones could suffer. When left untreated, it can cause irreversible damage to the bones. In addition, it can eventually cause issues in the blood vessels and the heart.

How Do We Combat This?

As we talked about a couple of chapters ago, your dietician will play an extremely important role in your health. He or she will examine your lab results along with the doctors and determine whether your levels of calcium and phosphorus are too high or too low and will adjust your diet to accommodate.

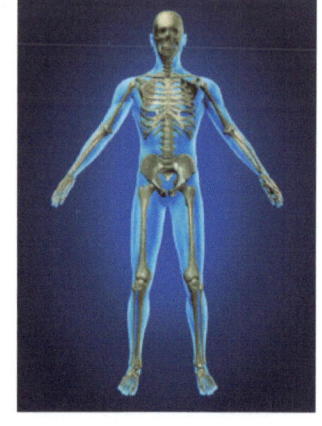

We pay an extraordinary amount of attention to your lab results so we can be sure you are on the right path to better health. We ensure that you get the replacement minerals you need to help maintain your bone health, as well as through medication. There needs to be a balance - you don't want the levels of calcium and phosphorous to be too low or too high. Our specialists are able to help strike this balance.

Chapter 10

Preventing Infections

Infection is a very serious topic, and it deserves its own chapter. If you have an infection, it can complicate treatment, and it can cause a number of other health problems. Many of the infections that patients get are staph infections, and this can cause issues with the heart valves. These types of infections often require a stay in the hospital, and the doctors will have to change out the catheter. Infection can increase the mortality of dialysis patients.

Catheters and Fistulas - Which Is Better?

Those patients who have catheters in place, both peritoneal and hemodialysis, will find that they are at a higher risk of infection if they do not take the proper precautions. One of the biggest dangers is getting them wet. This can quickly cause an infection.

As we talked about earlier, the fistulas are a much better option, so talk with your doctor about getting one of these instead. Fistulas have a lower risk of infection, but it can still happen. When you have a fistula, you will be able to get it wet without worry.

What Are the Signs and Symptoms of an Infection?

Let's look at some of the most common signs and symptoms of an infection:

- Increased pain
- Swelling or redness in the area
- Warmth around the site
- Drainage of puss from the site
- Fever

- Red streaks that extend from the site

What Can You Do?

When you are in the clinic, the nurse will provide you with instructions on how you can prevent infections. In addition, you can use the following tips.

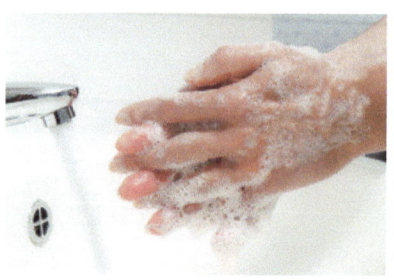

If you have a catheter, you have to make sure that you do not get it wet. In addition, you need to make sure you are washing your hands often, so you are not transferring any germs to the catheter when you touch it. You just need to make sure your hands are dry before you touch the catheter.

Always make sure you follow the steps provided by your healthcare professionals when it comes to using the catheter. In addition, make sure you know the signs and symptoms of infection so you are aware if you have any issues that need to be attended to by the doctor. Contact the doctor if you have a feeling there could be an infection. The earlier you catch it the better.

When it comes to a fistula or a graft, preventing infection is actually quite a bit easier. Make sure that you are taking proper care of the dialysis site per the information provided by the nurse. Again, you will want to wash your hands often. Clean the dialysis access site before and after treatment. As before, know the signs of infection and contact your doctor if you have any fears of infection.

Chapter 11

Networking with Other Patients

When you have chronic kidney disease and you are undergoing dialysis, having a strong support system is essential. You may have family and friends who have been great about supporting you during this time. However, that's not always 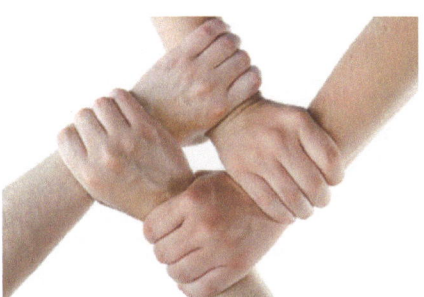 enough. Sometimes, you and your family would benefit greatly from networking with and befriending other patients who go to the clinic. It can actually provide you with a number of fantastic benefits.

You can find patients at the clinic when you are going through treatment, and you can find a number of patients through online networks, which we will discuss in a later chapter. In addition, you can talk with your social worker about these and other organizations that you can become a part of to meet and speak with other patients.

Let's look at a couple of those benefits now.

Talking About Life, Treatment, and More

First, it's always nice to meet new people and to become friends. However, when you are talking with other patients and their families, you are speaking with people who know exactly what you are going through and feeling. They've been through the same thing. Other friends you have, as supportive and sympathetic as they might be, do not truly understand what you are going through if they haven't experienced it themselves.

When you speak with others, you can also find out some information that the doctors and nurses don't tell you. It's not that the medical staff doesn't want to help; it's simply that the patients have a different perspective on things. For example, they can provide you with some ideas on what you can do during your treatment sessions, as we talked about earlier in the book.

One of the other nice things about speaking with and becoming friends with the other patients is that you can become friends with their family. Your family can discuss what life is like dealing with this new and difficult situation. Having others who understand can be extraordinarily helpful and can often be better than other types of therapy sessions that you might attend with your family.

Extracurricular Activities

You will also discover there are quite a few extracurricular activities you and the other patients can enjoy. Whether it's simply heading out for a day together, engaging in and training for Special Olympics competitions together, or even just getting together to cook and try out a new recipe you can enjoy plenty of things with one another. Think about some of the things that you enjoy doing and start making some plans.

Online Support

Keep in mind that you don't always have to meet with patients in person. As we touched on, there are plenty of online networks, and they can be a wonderful source of finding other patients in your area and around the rest of the country - and even other parts of the world!

Many of the sites have forums and message boards where you can communicate with one another. They tend to be very friendly places where everyone is encouraging and supportive.

You Will Feel Better

When you have more friends who understand what you are dealing with, it helps you to appreciate that you are not alone in your fight. It can help to combat depression and make you feel better overall. Just because you are on dialysis does not mean that you have to stop enjoying life. Networking with other patients will help you to make the most out of life.

Chapter 12

Traveling When You Are on Dialysis

Questions about travel are some of the most common that we get from patients and their family members. Many people love to travel, whether they are simply heading out of town for a weekend or going across the country, or even across the world 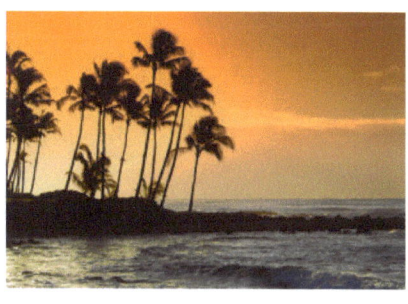 for a proper, long vacation. When they receive their diagnosis of chronic kidney disease and learn that they will need to go on dialysis, people fear that they will no longer be able to travel.

After all, if they are required to be on dialysis several times a week at a clinic, they feel that this will confine them to the area around the home for the rest of their life. Naturally, this can make patients feel depressed, almost as though they are living as shut-ins.

Fortunately, it's not true. You can actually travel even if you are a dialysis patient. Fresenius Dialysis has centers located all around the world and you can have access to them. In fact, we have a patient right now who loves to travel, and we've set up temporary dialysis in Hawaii, as well as other countries around the globe. All you need to do is speak with your social worker (see, we told you how helpful they are!) and they can set it up for you. Try to give us at least one to two week's notice so we can arrange the visit for you.

Now, what about patients who are using peritoneal dialysis at home? The cycler that you use is large and difficult to take with you while traveling. This doesn't mean you have to stay home though. We can set up an exchange while you are traveling. Your

PD nurse will be able to help you with this.

As you can see, no matter what type of dialysis you are on, you can still enjoy traveling with your family and friends. You just need to make sure you set things up with us far enough in advance to ensure everything works out smoothly.

Precautions While Traveling

While it is certainly possible to travel even though you need dialysis, and we highly encourage patients to get out and live their lives, we do urge you to take some precautions while you are doing so. In this section, we want to cover some of the basics you should keep in mind while you are traveling. As always, you should take the time to talk with your nurse, dietician, and doctor about other precautions you will need to take.

Keeping Clear of Infection

When you are traveling, there's a high likelihood that you will be exposed to far more germs than you would when you are around your house. This means that you have to be even more aware of your surroundings and the things that you are doing while you are on vacation. Stay away from areas that you believe would put you at a higher risk, and always take precautions when you are outside and around lots of people.

As always, you should make sure you wash your hands completely - and regularly - so that there is less of a risk of passing germs on from your hands to the fistula site. You might even want to take some hand sanitizer with you while you are out, just in case you don't have immediate access to soap and water.

Eating Right

When traveling, eating right and sticking to your diet can be somewhat difficult, even in the best of circumstances. Since you are on a specialized diet though, it can be even harder. It's extremely important that you stick to your diet though, so you should speak with your dietician before you travel. He or she can provide you with some suggestions on what you should do, and what you can eat, while you are away.

Spend a little bit more time looking at the menu so you can determine your best options, or even bring some food along with you on the vacation (or shop while you are there and cook on your own), so you can remain healthy and on your diet.

Plan Properly

As you can see, traveling, even though you need to go through dialysis, is very doable. You just need to start planning a little bit earlier. Think about where you will be going and what you will be doing, and make sure you schedule your vacation so that you can get to the dialysis appointments. Be wary of areas and activities that might increase your risk of infection, and have a plan in place when it comes to sticking to your diet. We can provide more suggestions on how you can have a safe and fun trip no matter where you decide to travel.

Chapter 13

When Should I Call the Doctor?

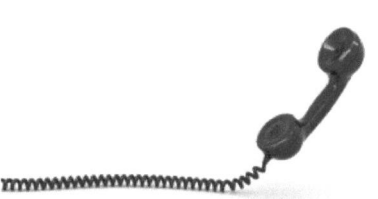

You are going through an entirely new experience when you are undergoing dialysis, and that means you do not always know when a problem is serious and you need to call the doctor, or when it is minor and normal. Well, I have to say that there is no such thing as a dumb question or concern, and if you ever have any worry, call us. Don't wait, don't hesitate, and don't think it will get better on its own. It is far better for your health that you get in touch with us so we can determine the nature and extent of the problem.

Make sure you have the phone numbers of your nephrologist and clinic saved in several locations. Have it written down at your home, and make sure you keep a list of these numbers conveniently located on your phone. This way, you will always have the numbers handy.

Top Reasons to Call the Doctor

Let's look at some of the reasons that you should contact the center immediately:

- Fever or Chills
- Bleeding Around the Catheter
- Pussy Discharge Around Catheter or Fistula
- Swelling, Redness, Tenderness at Dialysis Site
- Dizziness
- Whenever You Feel Concerned About a Complication or Health Issue

We don't believe there's any such thing as a small problem when it comes to your health. We understand the fear and questions that you will have whenever there is anything out of the ordinary, and we encourage you to call us so we can allay those fears or get you the help you need.

These are just some of the most common reasons that you will want to call your doctor or nurse. Every patient is different and may have a different set of questions or problems they notice after or before going through their treatment. We've mentioned this countless times before in this book, but I really believe it's important to repeat: always ask questions. After all, asking is the only way to get the answers you need.

Consider Your Medications

Often, the source of the issues people are having is directly related to the medications they are taking. It is a good idea that you bring along your pillbox to the center at least once a month, and whenever you have any changes to your medications. The nurse will check the medications to make sure you aren't taking duplicates, and that you have all of the correct meds. We've discovered that you can alleviate many complications that crop up simply by making sure you are taking the right medications in the right dosages.

In addition, before you start taking any over-the-counter medications, it is always a good idea to talk with your doctor and nurse, just to make sure that there will be no problems.

Chapter 14
Am I a Transplant Candidate?

Patients often wonder whether they are candidates for transplants. This is something that you will need to talk about with your physician. Your social worker at the clinic will be able to help you make the referral to a transplant center. Most of the time, the process of looking for potential transplants will begin as soon as you start dialysis. While your nurse and social worker will provide you with the full details on the process from start to finish, it's a good idea to have a basic idea of what to expect and how it works. We'll be covering that in this chapter.

How Does Transplanting Work?
When getting a transplant, you could receive a cadaveric kidney or a kidney from a living donor. It's important to understand the difference between the two. One of the most important differences is the timeframe for the transplant.

What Is a Cadaveric Kidney?
This is a kidney that you would receive from a donor who passes away. In most cases, finding a transplant can take between two and three years, although the exact timeframe is uncertain. In some cases, it is faster, and sometimes it may take longer to find a suitable donor. It may also be faster to find a donor in certain regions. Fortunately, it is possible for you to register in more than one region.

To determine whether you are a candidate for a transplant, you will need to undergo a number of different tests through cardiologists, gastroenterologists, dentists, and psychologists. Once you pass the exams, you will be put on the waiting list. When there is a kidney available, and your time is up on the list, you will be able to get your transplant.

A Living Donor

Some patients may not want to wait for a cadaveric kidney, or they may feel they do not have the time to wait. In those cases, it is possible to find a living donor. Humans have two kidneys, but we only need one to survive and be healthy. A living donor will provide you with one of his or her kidneys.

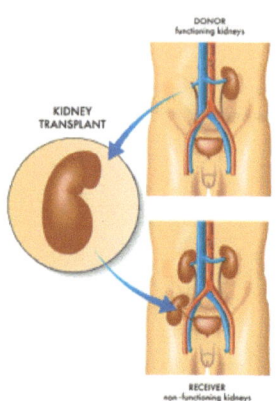

The process is much simpler, and when you have donors available, there is no waiting list. Most of the time, you will find two or three donors, and they will be tested for their blood group, and for HLA (human leukocyte antigen) matching. Once you find suitable donors, you can have a transplant in a relatively short period, so long as you are healthy enough.

Staying Healthy for the Transplant

Whether you are on the waiting list for a kidney, or you have a donor lined up, you need to make sure you do your best to stay as healthy as possible. If you are overweight, this means you will want to do your best to start losing weight. You can talk with your dietician about changing your diet to help you drop pounds, and you can speak with the doctor and nurses about exercises you can do to get into better shape. Being a proper weight and being healthy overall will increase the chance of the transplant being a success.

Always make sure you are taking your medications as prescribed, and make sure you do not miss any appointments with your healthcare team. If you have any changes in your health, make sure you let the transplant team know about them. When you are getting ready for a transplant, you can speak with your nephrologist about rejection medications, as well as the overall process and what you can expect.

Learn More

The goal of many people with chronic kidney disease is to

get a transplant and to have it be successful. Taking the time to understand the things you can in order to increase your chance of success could make a big difference. Make sure you ask your healthcare team about all of the things you can do.

Chapter 15

Special Olympics

While most associate the Special Olympics and similar organizations to be specifically for those who have intellectual disabilities, they encompass far more than that. They have games available for those who have many other types of disabilities and handicaps as well, including those who are on dialysis.

If you are interested in learning more and competing in these or other types of games, you can speak with your social worker. They can provide you with all of the details you need about the games and how to enter. As we mentioned, you can also speak with other patients who are going through dialysis. Some of them may have participated in various types of athletic competitions, and they could have some good information about how you can join as well.

You can find a number of different organizations, including the Renal Network, which we will discuss in Chapter 19. They often arrange different types of activities for patients, as well as for their family members.

Let's look at a few of the types of activities you may be able to enjoy:

- Equestrian
- Tennis
- Powerlifting
- Roller Skating
- Bowling
- Cycling
- Table Tennis

These are just a few of the potential activities offered through the Special Olympics as well as other organizations. You can find plenty of other options out there. Find some activities you enjoy and then consider participating. It can be quite a bit of fun, especially when you have friends competing with you or against you!

How Can Participating Help You?

When you are first diagnosed with chronic kidney disease and find out you need to go on dialysis, thinking about partaking in athletic activities is probably the last thing on your mind. You have a lot on your mind, and it can feel overwhelming. This book, along with the help you can receive from the doctors, nurses, social workers, dieticians and the rest of the staff should help you to get a better grasp of your situation though. At that point, it is important that you take the time to start doing things for yourself that you enjoy, and these types of games and activities can bring you quite a bit of happiness and joy.

Getting more exercise training for the games and participating can be a huge benefit for your health. It can help you keep your weight down and your spirits high. When you exercise, it releases endorphins into the body that simply make you feel great. Competing, getting to know the other competitors, and simply spending more time with family and friends can make a difference.

If you are thinking about participating, make sure you talk with your doctor first to make sure that you are healthy enough to exercise and compete in the sports that you would like. We want you to get out there and have fun, but we want you to be safe as well.

Chapter 16

Do You Have High Cholesterol?

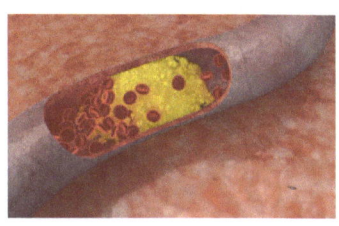

When you are on dialysis, your body is undergoing a large amount of stress. Some patients have high blood pressure, which can make dialysis more difficult. It can also increase the risk of developing heart disease and it is actually common with those who already have chronic kidney disease. Having high cholesterol can complicate matters further. We take cholesterol very seriously at the clinic, and we will be checking it every three months. The doctor will go over the results with you and will help you make adjustments so you can get it down to normal levels.

People who have chronic kidney disease are more prone to having issues with narrowing blood vessels. High cholesterol will exacerbate this problem, so maintaining proper levels of cholesterol in the body is highly important.

What Is Cholesterol?

Humans get cholesterol from two different sources. It is produced naturally by the liver and it is ingested through the foods that we eat. Some of the types of foods that have the highest levels of cholesterol include eggs, dairy foods, seafood, and meat. It is not possible to control the amount of cholesterol that the body produces naturally. However, it is possible to control what we eat, and that's where the dietician comes into play. We'll discuss that further in the next section. For now, let's get an understanding for "good" and "bad" cholesterol.

Bad cholesterol, or LDL, creates plaque on the arteries. This is a thick deposit on the walls, and it reduces the flow of blood and makes the arteries less flexible. The term for this is atherosclerosis. In some cases, when a clot forms, it can cause a heart attack or a stroke.

Good cholesterol is HDL cholesterol and it can actually help to remove the LDL cholesterol in the arteries. It is believed that it carries the LDL back to the liver, where it will break it down so it can be passed through the body. Higher HDL may also help to provide protection from heart attack and stroke. In fact, having low levels of HDL can actually increase the risk of heart disease. The desirable levels of good and bad cholesterol in the blood can vary based on a number of reasons. You can speak with your doctor about the ideal levels as well as the things that you should do to attain them.

Your Dietician Can Help

The dietician understands the importance of limiting cholesterol in your diet, and he or she will factor this into creating your diet plan. By adjusting the diet so that you have better overall foods and you are ingesting less LDL and more HDL, it is possible to start to get the cholesterol under control naturally. Your dietician will work with you to make sure that your cholesterol stays under control.

As mentioned, we have monthly meetings where we go over labs. Controlling cholesterol is an important part of this, and we work together to provide you with the best possible outcome.

Medications

If you have high cholesterol and are like many patients out there, you likely take medications to help. When you are starting dialysis, it might be necessary to adjust these medications. We'll be monitoring your cholesterol and can adjust the meds as needed.

Tips to Help

Let's look at a couple of simple tips that you can employ to help you keep your blood vessels in shape and to keep high cholesterol at bay. First, if you are a smoker, you need to stop. You already know that smoking is extremely unhealthy and can cause cancer and heart disease. Did you know that it could speed up disease and damage in blood vessels as well?

If you are overweight, try to lose weight. The dietician can help with this, but you will want to try to get some exercise as well. Just make sure you speak with the doctor to make sure you are healthy enough for exercise.

Take steps to control your blood pressure, and ask the doctor about any medications that might help, if you are not already on meds for your high cholesterol. Do not start taking any over-the-counter medications such as aspirin to thin the blood without first consulting with your doctor.

Chapter 17

Working and Dialysis

If you are on dialysis, you are probably wondering how you will be able to keep your job. We've already talked about how important it is to make sure you do what you can to maintain your lifestyle and as much of your social life as possible. However, work is another matter. You want to keep working. Chances are you are like most people out there and you need to keep working. It is very important that you have your medical insurance, and you should be able to keep it even if you go on temporary disability.

What Can Employers Do to Help?

Fortunately, most employers are accommodating. You need to know what you can and can't do at your job and let them know. For example, many people who have chronic kidney disease and who go through dialysis will feel tired faster than they did in the past. 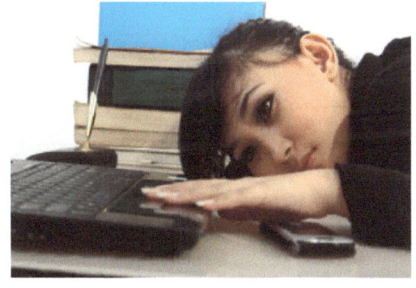 However, that's not always the case. The employer will often be able to make certain concessions and change up some of your job responsibilities. Talk with your employer about what they might be able to change with your job to accommodate you. Make sure they understand the appointments you may have through the week for your dialysis as well.

At Fresenius, we understand how important it is for you to keep working, and we'll do our best to help you. You can work with your social worker to help you with this, and your doctor can write a letter of support for you.

Patients often worry that after they've gone through dialysis, they will be too weak and wiped out to work. That is not always the case. In fact, we've found that most of the patients feel fine after their dialysis session, and they are able to go to work immediately. Of course, in some patients, such as those who have comorbid conditions, there is more of a weakness after they've gone through dialysis. They may need to rest after they've gone through their dialysis procedure. The vast majority of people will be able to keep their job though.

Keep in mind that it will often depend on the type of work that you do. In some cases, there will be physical things that you normally do that are no longer possible, or that might not be safe for you. In those cases, you can speak with your employer about ways that you may be able to transition to another position at the company.

Support You Need

You can work with your social worker to get the support you need when you are talking with your employer, but that's not the only support out there for you. The social worker can help you connect to organizations such as the American Kidney Fund and the Renal Network. They have a number of resources that can help to make your life easier, and we'll cover these in detail later in the book. For example, the American Kidney Fund, along with your dialysis clinic, can help to make sure you are able to maintain your medical insurance.

Getting in touch and being active with these organizations can offer support for more than just your work life though, as we'll discuss later. They could become some of the most important groups in your life.

Don't Give Up on the Idea of Working

Just because you are on dialysis, it does not mean that you are not able to work. It only means that you will need to adjust your work life in certain ways. With the support and help that we offer, it should be possible to continue working and living your life as normally as possible.

Chapter 18

Family Fatigue

So far, we've discussed what living with chronic kidney disease and going through dialysis can mean to you. However, your family is also a part of this journey, and it is extremely important to remember what they are going through as well. Not only are they worried about you, but they are also helping in a number of different ways when it comes to providing you support.

How Does the Family Help?

For example, if you are not active and you aren't able to drive, they will be responsible for providing transportation for you to and from the dialysis center, as well as for all of the other places that you have to go. They will often be helping with many of your other daily activities as well. They might even help to make sure you are taking the right medications - this is actually common with many older patients. If you are doing dialysis at home, chances are good that they are helping you with these procedures as well.

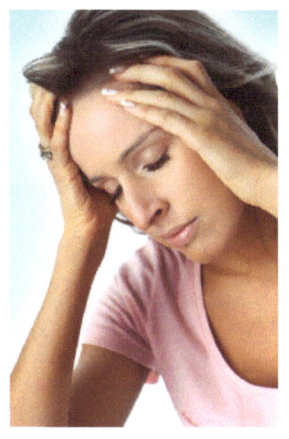

You are eternally grateful for the love, support, and help they are able to offer. However, if they don't have a break, it can lead to fatigue and a buildup of stress. They have plenty of things that they have to do to take care of themselves as well, and relying on only one or two people for the help you need is not ideal.

Even in those cases where there are multiple family members willing to help, often they all try to do everything at the same time. It's nice to have that support, but they really should take turns and divvy up the work. If they don't, there's a chance that they could run into something called family fatigue, and the stress will build up in them.

What Are the Signs of Family Fatigue and Stress?

Some of the most common signs and symptoms that the family is getting stressed and burned out include:

- Depression
- Anxiety
- Irritability
- Insomnia
- Health Problems
- Trouble Concentrating
- Neglecting Other Responsibilities
- No Longer Engaging in Leisure Activities

Let's look at a few ways that you can avoid this and how the family can remove their stress.

Tips for Removing Stress

One of the first things that you and the family should do is to sit down and think about the type of help you need and when. Which family members will be best suited for different tasks, and when will they be available. Then, you can create a schedule so that they can accommodate your needs and still have time for themselves. When you are making the schedule, make sure that everyone is being honest about how much time is available as well as how they can help. You don't want to overburden anyone, and you don't want to be relying on them for help only to find out later that they aren't able to be there for you.

You will find that having a schedule where everyone knows what is expected can relieve a substantial amount of stress. It's not the only way though.

Family members should do their best to remain as active as possible when it comes to their social life and their health. Getting out with friends, exercising, and meditating can all be fantastic ways to reduce stress and to make it easier to deal with real life problems. Eating well and getting plenty of sleep can help as well.

In some cases, family members might want to speak with family members of other patients to see how they handle things. They could also meet with a local or online support group.

Make sure you speak with your nurse and social worker about some of the other things you and your family can do as a means to reduce the risk of family fatigue. We know that it's a tough time for everyone in the family, and we want to make sure you get through it intact. The important thing is that you and your family take action and are proactive against these sorts of issues.

Chapter 19

Dealing with Depression

As people reach the end stage of renal disease and they have to go on dialysis, it is natural for feelings of depression to set in, given the changes they need to make to their lifestyle. With some patients, the feelings leave as soon as they start to learn more about the process of dialysis as well as what they can expect. However, that's not always the case. Sometimes, the depression lasts and simply won't go away. If you are having these feelings, it is extremely important that you seek help.

Depression is preventable, and it is possible to pull out of a depressive state. Some may be in a depressive state without even realizing it. Depression has a number of different symptoms. You and your family will want to watch for some of the following signs and symptoms.

Signs of Depression

Here's a quick list of some of the most common signs of being depressed.

- Perpetual feelings of sadness, even when the same activities would normally make you feel happy
- Irritability
- Difficulty making decisions
- Changes in sleep patterns - more sleep or less sleep than usual
- Constant feeling of being tired
- Changes in appetite - eating more or less than normal
- Constant thoughts of death - when this occurs, you need to contact help immediately

What Can You Do About Depression?

If you find that you are in the throes of depression, you need to do your best to get help and to make changes in your life. You should speak with your doctor, as well as the dialysis nurse and the social worker at the clinic. Your social worker can help you find resources to give the help needed. Now is the time to rely on your spouse or significant other, as well as a trusted friend. If you are religious, you can speak with your religious leader for some guidance.

Those who are feeling depressive enough that they are thinking about suicide should rethink the situation. Contact the suicide hotline by calling 1-800-SUICIDE. If it is an emergency and you are contemplating harming yourself, or if you have harmed yourself, contact 911 immediately. You have people who love you, and they want you to be around for as long as possible.

In some cases, the doctor or nurse practitioner will prescribe medication that can help with your depressed state. You may also want to speak with a psychiatrist who can help you through these feelings. If the psychiatrist is going to prescribe a medication for you, it is extremely important that you speak with your nephrologist to make sure the medications will not react negatively with one another. There could be a need to change the dosages.

You may also want to consider some psychotherapy sessions, where you can talk through your feelings. In some cases, your employer may even have a program that you can use, and it could be covered by your insurance. Other help could be available through the department of social services in your county.

The point of this chapter is to let you know that depression is entirely treatable. You can do plenty of things, so do not let being depressed rule you.

Chapter 20

American Kidney Fund and Renal Network

As we talked about several times earlier in the book, a number of organizations are dedicated to helping patients who are going through the same thing that you are right now. Two of the most prominent are the American Kidney Fund and the Renal Network. In this chapter, we are going to take a closer look at each of these organizations and will provide you with information on how to get in touch with them. If you want to know more about how they might be able to help you, make sure that you speak with your nurse or social worker.

The American Kidney Fund

The American Kidney Fund is a fantastic resource for patients. They strive to make sure that all patients have access to healthcare, and that they receive the education they need to make the most of their life. They also act as advocates for patients. In the last year alone, the AKF was able to provide financial assistance to about 20% of the dialysis patients in the United States.

This is a massive help. Perhaps you have been having trouble affording all of the medications you are taking. If not, then you probably know someone else who is struggling now or who has struggled in the past. It is nice to have an organization out there that works for and advocates for patients such as you.

They have a number of programs to help patients in a variety of ways. The HelpLine provides answers about your kidneys, dialysis, the meaning of your diagnosis, and more. It's a good resource for patients, as well as for family members who have questions. They also have programs for children who are kidney patients, including those that offer summer enrichment activities, art contests, and more. One of the other great benefits of the AKF is their prescription drug resources that can help people who don't have insurance for medicines and who can't afford them.

The best way to get in touch with the American Kidney Fund is to go directly to their website (www.KidneyFund.Org), or to write to them at the following address to get more information:

American Kidney Fund
11921 Rockville Pike, Suite 300
Rockville, MD 20852

The Renal Network

The Renal Network is a not-for-profit organization with the task of monitoring the quality of dialysis care in various states. The goal is to promote high quality care for patients, and they offer a number of services for patients.

The Patient Services Department will investigate patient complaints and concerns, provide coating for staff and patients, and created educational resources for patients. One of their primary goals is to connect patients. They've found that patients who know a lot about their condition tend to have better outcomes and outlooks. Connecting patients so they can share this knowledge has been extremely helpful.

To contact them, you can visit their website (www.therenalnetwork.org). The website is full of useful information. They have tools and resources that cover fistulas, mental health of patients, rights and responsibilities, and much more. There is a substantial amount of information on the site, and it might not all pertain directly to you. You will still want to explore everything they offer though.

Talk With the Social Worker

Do you want to know more about these and other organizations for kidney and dialysis patients? Your social worker is one of the best resources for you. They can provide you with contact information, tips on making the most of these organizations, and much more.

Chapter 21

Getting Help with Prescription Costs

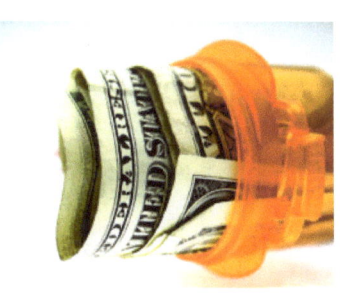

Many people find that the cost of their prescriptions can end up putting them in the hold financially before they know it. When you are on dialysis, you might also be suffering from other comorbid conditions that would require you to start taking more medications. As you know, this simply compounds the costs. Some types of prescriptions, particularly binders and blood pressure medications, are extremely costly, and you could find that your insurance simply can't cover everything.

What Should You Do?

You can't go without your medications. Your health is on the line and you need to find ways that you can get the medication you need. If you stop taking the medications, or if you try to lower your dosages on your own, it could end up causing far more complications that can harm your health even further. We understand the struggle you are going through right now.

Fortunately, we may be able to provide you with some guidance and help in this area. For example, you might find that your doctor is able to get you some samples, which can help to lower your expenditure, as you will not have to buy as much medication. However, this tends to be a temporary fix.

Your social worker is going to be a huge benefit to you, and could be the answer to your problems. They will be able to help you get into prescription drug programs and they can put you into contact with patient access networks to help you get the medications that you need. In the last chapter, we covered the American Kidney Fund. They are a fantastic resource that has been helping patients such as you get access to the medications they need.

Tips for Saving on Your Medication

You have a number of other options when it comes to potentially saving on the cost of your medication. Talk with your doctor about the drugs you are taking and ask if there are generic options that you could be taking instead. They work the same, but they are generally quite a bit cheaper. This can help to lower your costs by quite a bit. While you might not be able to find generics for all of your meds right now, chances are you will have a generic option for quite a few of them.

In addition, it could be a good idea to start looking at other insurance options. You might actually find that it is cheaper to go with a higher-level insurance program that covers more of the cost of prescriptions. Even though you might be paying more for the insurance, it could still be cheaper when you calculate the cost of your medications if you didn't have the insurance.

Be proactive in looking for ways that you can save on your prescription costs. It will help you in the end.

Chapter 22

Frequently Asked Questions

We've tried to answer a number of the common questions that people have when it comes to dialysis thus far in the book. In this chapter, we'll be looking at some of the most common questions, including some we've covered, just so we can have them all in one place and answer them nicely and succinctly.

Common Questions

What Is Chronic Kidney Disease?

Chronic kidney disease is a condition that causes the gradual loss of kidney function over a period. The speed with which the shutdown occurs will vary based on a number of factors. It is far more common than many people realize. In fact, around 26 million people in the United States alone have chronic kidney disease. Many of these people will need to go through dialysis as they kidneys slowly lose functionality.

What Is Dialysis?

Dialysis is needed when a patient is reaching the end stage of kidney failure. This will usually occur when around 85% to 90% of the kidney function stops. The dialysis treatment, whether opting for hemodialysis or peritoneal dialysis, helps to remove the waste from the body, along with removing extra salt and water. It ensures there is a safe level of chemicals in the body, and it can even help to control blood pressure.

Is Kidney Failure Permanent?

This is a very common question among patients. Unfortunately, you will find that in the majority of cases, kidney failure is permanent. However, that's not always the case. Sometimes, acute kidney failure can improve after treatment and dialysis may only be needed for a short time. Those who have chronic kidney failure though will find that their kidneys will not improve and will need to be on dialysis for the rest of their life, or will need to get a transplant.

How Long Does a Transplanted Kidney Work?

If you are eligible for a transplant, you likely want to know how long one of these transplants will actually be able to last. Today, the success rate of transplants is actually very high. Once you have a new working kidney in the body, the length of time it lasts depends on a number of factors. Those who have a cadaveric kidney will find that it could last between 10 and 15 years. Those who receive a kidney from a live donor could have it last up to 20 years or more in some cases. However, part of this will be dependent on how well you take care of your body.

Can I Drive After Dialysis?

After a dialysis treatment, nothing can actually stop you from driving. It's not against the law. In fact, many people drive themselves to and from the appointments for treatment. However, you have to remember that there is always the potential for some danger, and some people should not be behind the wheel. If you find that the treatments make you feel weak and lower your blood pressure, then avoid driving. Have someone else take you. If you can, schedule your treatment at a time of day when you can avoid the bulk of the traffic on the way home.

What Can I Eat?

When you have chronic kidney disease and are on dialysis, your diet is extremely important to your health. Just trying to eat healthy is not enough. You need to make sure you listen to your dietician and pay attention to their eating and nutrition guidelines. You can still eat many of the foods you love, but you want to make sure that you are abiding by their rules.

What If I Miss Dialysis?

You do not want to miss your dialysis treatment if you can

help it. The dialysis is the only way your body is able to remove waste and contaminants, and if you miss dialysis, it could cause a number of other health problems in a relatively short period. It is possible to miss an appointment without a problem, but you do not want to miss two appointments in a row. You should never try to go more than three days without a treatment. It is dangerous. If you feel as though you might miss a treatment, call the clinic so you can reschedule as soon as possible.

How Long Does Dialysis Take?

On average, it will take four hours to complete dialysis treatment. However, the exact time can vary based on the patient. This is something that you will want to discuss with your doctor and nurse. Once you've had one treatment, you will know how long it should take to complete. It tends to be the same from session to session.

Is Dialysis Uncomfortable?

Most patients will not feel any real discomfort when they are going through their treatments. There could be a slight amount of discomfort when the needles are added to the graft or fistula, but this is minor and temporary. The actual treatment does not cause any pain at all. Some patients could experience a drop in their blood pressure though, which could cause nausea or even cramps. As you go through more and more treatments though, these symptoms tend to disappear.

Should I Keep Working?

This is often up to you, as well as how you feel after treatments. Most patients find that they feel fine enough to work after they go through dialysis. They have no trouble getting back to work. Other patients may not want to work if they are going on dialysis. It's important to consider how you feel, as well as the reality of your finances, to determine whether you should keep working. If you haven't checked out our chapter on working, go back and read it now.

What Can the Family Do to Help?

Your family will be one of your primary sources of support when you have chronic kidney disease. They will often help with transportation, helping you run errands, and helping with some basic tasks.

How Much Longer Will I Live?

This question is difficult, and nearly impossible to answer since each patient is different. You will need to continue with your dialysis treatments for the remainder of your life. The average life expectancy is between five and 10 years. However, there have been patients who have lived on dialysis for much longer. To get a better idea of your life expectancy, you need to speak with your doctor and not merely base your information on averages though.

Chapter 23

Becoming a Star Patient

In our clinic, we work hard to make sure you always know what's happening with each of our patients' health. We perform labs, compare meds, check the charts, and set up goals for all of our patients each month. Everything that we do is in an effort to improve the outcome of our patients. We work hard, but that doesn't mean that you are off the hook!

If you want to become a star patient and have the best possible outcome, it means you need to participate in the clinic programs and follow them. You need to work as hard toward being healthy as we do.

Don't worry; it's simple, and it is everything that we've already covered. Make sure you are there for your treatments a little bit early. You need to make certain you are taking your medications properly, and that you are following your diet and the guidelines recommended by your doctor and dietician.

When you follow the course of action we prescribe, everyone wins. You will get healthier and we'll be proud of your achievements. As you can see, it's actually easy to become one of our star patients!

Chapter 24

Do I Need Handicap Parking?

This is actually a very common question so I thought we would address it in its own short chapter.

Is It Necessary?

So, do you need to have handicap parking now that you are going on dialysis? In most cases, no, you don't. As we talked about earlier in the book, many people who are on dialysis feel fine after they go through the procedure. Most are even able to go right back to work. This means 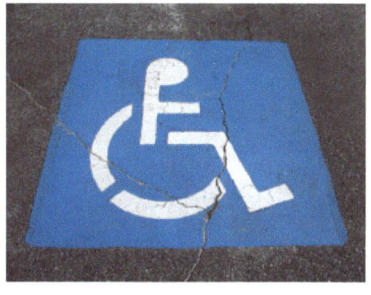 that you probably do not need to have handicap parking.

In fact, some people feel self-conscious about getting a handicap sticker for their vehicle when they have kidney disease since it is a disease that people can't "see". You aren't in a wheelchair, and you might worry about people not believing that you are handicapped when you roll into a spot. If you don't feel as though you really need a sticker, then there is no reason to get one.

However, if you find that you are getting too tired while you are walking around, or that you feel short of breath or weak, then it is actually a good idea to consider a handicap-parking permit.

Getting the Permit

If you feel that you do need to have one of these permits, it's important to remember that the rules vary in different locations. You will want to make sure that you speak with your social worker about what you need to do in order to get your permit. You will need an application and will need to go through the motor vehicle department. You could request a permanent or a temporary placard. You can get a placard or license plates. Most opt to use the placard, as it will allow you to use it in any vehicle you are in or driving.

Don't Feel Ashamed

This can be difficult to get across to many patients who have kidney disease and who are undergoing dialysis. Many like to keep their illness hidden, and others don't want people staring at them and wondering why they have a parking placard since there does not appear to be anything wrong with them. If you need one, never feel ashamed about using it. Those people who you feel are judging you are not as important as your health. Please keep this in mind when you are debating about whether you should use the placard or not.

Chapter 25

My Nurse Was Rude!

When you are coming into the clinic for a treatment or any other reason, the last thing you want to deal with is a nurse or any staff member who you feel treats you rudely or poorly. There is no excuse for this type of behavior from any staff member, but there is always the possibility that something such as this could happen. People may not be having a good day. They may have had to deal with a number of problems, and they might be at their wit's end.

What Happened?

Sure, they are all human, and that means that there could be days where they seem distant or rude. It might seem as though they are not listening and that they ignore you. Still, there's no excuse for this. One of the things that I've always stressed with everyone on the staff is that they need to take extra care with the patient's needs. They've been trained to listen to the patient and to get an understanding of what they need and to do everything they can to meet those needs.

We've found that bad employees do not last long here. We find them and we get rid of them. We really do want the best for you, and that includes a caring and compassionate staff. Earlier in the book, I mentioned that the staff and patients have a familial relationship with one another. That's something that we strive to maintain. It helps to build a much stronger support system for you.

If you truly feel as if they were rude to you, or that they are not listening to you, you have the right to speak with a nurse manager or social worker. They will make sure that your needs are attended to. There is no reason and no excuse for the staff to be rude to the patients, or to one another for that matter.

Fortunately, we are quite proud of our staff and we do our best to hire only high quality, empathetic individuals who want the best for the patients, and we believe that you will truly enjoy your interactions with everyone on the team.

Chapter 26

Learning the Lingo - Your Quick and Simple Glossary

When you first receive your diagnosis, chances are good that you will start to hear quite a few terms that are unfamiliar to you. As we've said plenty of other times, you should feel free to ask questions whenever you are uncertain. However, I also thought it would be handy to provide you with a nice and simply glossary that you can refer to as a means to get information on some of the most common words and phrases you will hear.

- **Binders** - These are phosphate binders, and they help to lower the phosphorous levels in the body. They are available in a number of different types of pills and capsules. Some of the most popular options include Tums, PhosLo, Renvela, and Velphoro. Your doctor and dietician will check your phosphorous levels regularly to determine what you need. These pills are often expensive, and your social worker can help you find ways to obtain them through different programs.

- **Shunt** - Also called a graft or fistula, this is one of the most common terms you will hear in the clinic. As we've stated before, these are far more preferable than using a catheter, as they tend to work better and clot less. The staff may refer to both of the accesses - fistula and catheter - as a shunt.

- **Sensipar** - This is a type of medicine used for bone and mineral metabolism, and it is often used by the dietician when talking about improvement for PTH levels, as well as calcium and phosphorous levels.

- **Protein** - Before starting dialysis, it is common for patients to need to cut down on their protein intake. Once starting dialysis, the opposite holds true. It is important that you eat plenty of protein, and your dietician will be able to help you with this substantially. Once you have some great recipes that you like, consider sharing them at the clinic. In general, we like our patients to eat between 60 and 100 grams of protein each day in many different varieties.

• **Catheter** - This is one type of dialysis access point, and we've already talked about it being the lesser method. They are more prone to infections when used for dialysis. Our goal is to have zero catheters in our clinic, and one bit of advice that I hope you take is that you should get rid of your catheter and get a fistula or graft as soon as possible. It is simply a better and safer option that can improve dialysis and even help you live longer.

• **Dry Weight** - As mentioned, you will be weighed before and after dialysis during each session. We have a large scale where you can weigh yourself. The weight after you've gone through dialysis, after removing extra fluid, is your dry weight, and it is measured in kilograms rather than pounds (1kg is 2.2 pounds). Make sure you remember this number - write it down. We try to adjust your post dialysis weight so that you have no extra fluid and so you feel good.

• **Weight Gain** - If you retain fluid, this could be a term that you hear often. We expect that our patients will not gain more than 1kg per day, but if you retain fluids, you could hear this term quite often. You will need to watch the amount of fluid that you take into the body, as well as your sodium intake. Eating salt tends to lead to more water retention and weight gain, which you do not want.

• **Cramps** - During the last half hour of dialysis, you might have cramps in your legs. This is common for many patients. The nurse can change your dry weight to help with this. If you are suffering from cramps, be sure you let the dialysis nurse know right away. The nurse can adjust the machines to help you.

• **It's Too Cold Here** - We mentioned that it can be a bit cool in the clinic, and you might hear this phrase from a number of patients. Bring a blanket. Most of the clinics will have a blanket that you can use, so you do not need to bring one along with you. If you are still too cold, let the nurse know and we'll see what we can do to accommodate you.

- **Hemoglobin, Iron, Epo or Micera** - Your hemoglobin will need to be at a certain level. We will provide an IV or epogen hormone to help with this. Some patients will also be provided iron through an IV as well. What you receive depends on the blood work, as well as what you need. In some cases, we will administer Micera, a new medication that can help with your hemoglobin. If you have any questions about the medications used, just ask.

- **Potassium Bath** - There are different types of potassium baths, which are settings on the dialysis machine. For example, if you have high potassium you would be on a low potassium bath and vice versa.

- **Adequacy** - This term is a measure of the amount of dialysis you are getting, and it is based on your monthly blood work. On the monthly report, you may hear words such as urea clearance and Kt/V, which can help the doctor determine your adequacy. The doctor or nurse may need to make changes to the machine, or they may look at your shunt or increase the amount of time you are on dialysis.

- **Dialyzer/Filter** - Each patient will have a different dialyzer used with dialysis. We use disposable dialyzers at Fresenius. If you hear the staff talking about an artificial kidney, chances are good they are talking about your dialyzer/filter.

- **24-Hour Urine** - Your doctor might ask you about your 24-hour urine collection. The nurse will provide you with medication and instructions on how you can collect it. In some cases, this happens in conjunction with the labs, so you can get a better idea of how the kidneys are working.

- **Exit Site Infection** - This is more common if you are on peritoneal dialysis or if you have a catheter. The skin around the catheter has a chance of developing an infection. We want to take care of the problem before the infection gets into the blood. Your nurse will let you know how to take care of the catheter properly.

• **Peritonitis** - Patients who are on peritoneal dialysis may suffer from peritonitis, which is an infection in the abdominal cavity. It is quite rare, and you can reduce the risk with proper hand washing and hygiene. We will educate you on taking care of the site, and we will draw cultures from the peritoneal fluid if necessary.

Conclusion

Now that we've come to the end of this book, I hope that you have a much better understanding of what it means to have chronic kidney disease and to be on dialysis. I hope you feel more comfortable when it comes to visiting the clinic and speaking with the staff, and I truly hope you've learned that it doesn't mean you have to stop doing everything that you love. You can still live and enjoy life.

When you understand more about the complexities of dialysis and all of the other elements of treatment you will be going through including things such as your diet, it can be much easier to handle the stress of this new situation.

Yes, there is still fear and there is still stress. However, this book has shown you ways to deal with these things in a constructive manner. Ask those questions. Be willing to make real changes in your life to improve your outcome. When you do, you will live longer and you will feel better.

I wish you all the best and everyone at the clinic looks forward to working with you!

About the Author

Deepak Mittal, MD is a board certified nephrologist currently practicing in Northren, Kentucky. He is also board certified in internal medicine. Dr. Mittal specializes in patients with End Stage Renal Disease and management of dialysis.

Dr. Mittal's current positions include:

- Medical Director for Fresenius Medical Care
- CEO and President of Kidney Disease Consultants
- Chief of Staff for Gateway Rehabilitation Center
- Assistant Professor of Medicine and Nephrology at A.T. Still University
- Medical Director for DSI Renal, Inc.
- Staff Nephrologist for KUMAR Dialysis
- Medical Director for Hillsboro Dialysis and SunBridge Healthcare
- Nephrologist at Highland District Hospital and St. Elizabeth Healthcare

Dr. Mittal's extensive education includes the University of Louisville School of Medicine for Nephorology and Internal Medicine, as well as the All India Institute of Medical Sciences, Government Medical College Patiala, and Government Ranbir College of Sangrur.

www.ingramcontent.com/pod-product-compliance
Lightning Source LLC
Chambersburg PA
CBHW040905180526
45159CB00010BA/2934